Kiesha L. Gayles- Author

Cover Letter:

This is a book for all to enjoy. This book covers all diet secrets and flaws to loosing weight.

The author Kiesha Gayles has created this book due to the world views on skinny is better and bigger is bad business.

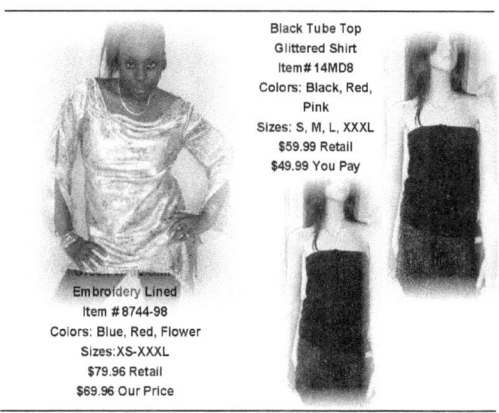

Black Tube Top
Glittered Shirt
Item# 14MD8
Colors: Black, Red, Pink
Sizes: S, M, L, XXXL
$59.99 Retail
$49.99 You Pay

Embroidery Lined
Item # 8744-98
Colors: Blue, Red, Flower
Sizes:XS-XXXL
$79.96 Retail
$69.96 Our Price

Diet secrets to lose weight fast!
(Have American's become too lazy?)
Guide to a safe way to lose weight

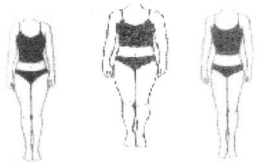

By: Kiesha Gayles
Editor: Charles Moore
Published By: Lulu.com

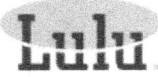

Author: Kiesha L. Gayles
Editor: Charles Moore

Published By: Lulu.com / Kiessand & Cam Co.

Special thanks: To Lulu.com and family my little sis Nicole and brothers
Charles and Mark and my son Cam.
Cam I would not be who I am if you were not born. I am trying to be beyond what I can
be for you. I love you.

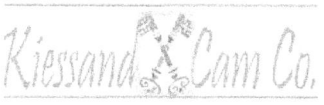

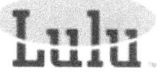

Chapters

Starving Yourself 4

Steps to relieve stress......................5

Thyroid Problem............................7

What a Man Wants.......................8

Types Of Diets............................11

Endorphins................................17

Things To Consider....................19

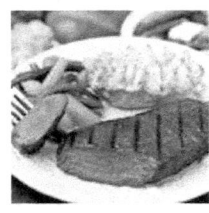

Starving Yourself

Many Americans think that the best way to lose weight is to starve themselves. The bread and water diet is not effective. Well it does help to a certain extent, like the image of looking like you smoke crack and major health problems. Like Anorexia, Bilema, etc.

ANOREXIA AND BULIMIA

What Is Anorexia?

Anorexia is an eating disorder where people starve themselves. Anorexia usually begins in young people around the onset of puberty. Individuals suffering from anorexia have extreme weight loss. Weight loss is usually 15% below the person's normal body weight. People suffering from anorexia are very skinny but are convinced that they are overweight. Weight loss is obtained by many ways. Some of the common techniques used are excessive exercise, intake of laxatives and not eating.

Anorexics have an intense fear of becoming fat. Their dieting habits develop from this fear. Anorexia mainly affects adolescent girls.

People with anorexia continue to think they are overweight even after they become extremely thin, are very ill or near death. Often they will develop strange eating habits such as refusing to eat in front of other people. Sometimes the individuals will prepare big meals for others while refusing to eat any of it.

The disorder is thought to be most common among whites, people of higher socioeconomic classes, and people involved in activities where thinness is especially looked upon, such as dancing, theater, and distance running.

A Family Member has an Eating Disorder

If you have a family member that with an Eating Disorder, they need a lot of support. Suggest that your family member see an eating disorder expert. Be prepared for denial, resistance, and even anger. A doctor and/or a counselor can help them battle their eating disorder.

Symptoms?

There are many symptoms for anorexia; some individuals may not experience all of them symptoms. The symptoms include: Body weight that is inconsistent with age, build and height (usually 15% below normal weight).

Some other symptoms are:

- Loss of at least 3 consecutive menstrual periods (in women).
- Not wanting or refusing to eat in public.
- Other symptoms are: anxiety, weakness, brittle skin, shortness of breath, obsessive ness about calorie intake

Medical Consequences?

There are many medical risks associated with anorexia. They include: shrunken bones, mineral loss, low body temperature, irregular heartbeat, permanent failure of normal growth, development of osteoporosis and bulimia nervosa.

Continued use of laxatives is harmful to the body. It wears out the bowel muscle and causes it to decrease in function. Some laxatives contain harsh substances that may be reabsorbed into your system.

Anorexia and Pregnancy

In order to have a healthy child, the average pregnant woman should gain between 25 and 35 pounds. Telling this to a person with anorexia is like telling a normal person to gain 100 pounds. If you are anorexic, you may have trouble conceiving a baby and carrying it to term. Irregular menstrual cycles and weak bones make it more difficult to conceive. If you are underweight and do not eat the proper variety of foods, you and your baby could be in danger.

Women with eating disorders have higher rates of miscarriages and your baby might be born prematurely which puts them at risk for many medical problems.

All pregnant women should receive proper prenatal care. Those recovering from anorexia or bulimia need special care. You should always take your pre-natal vitamins and have regular pre-natal visits. You should not exercise unless your doctor says it is okay and it is a good idea to enroll in a prenatal exercise class to be sure you are not overexerting yourself.

If you have anorexia or bulimia, you can stop it in its tracks by enrolling in a treatment program and eating and exercising in healthy ways. You can also learn to reduce stress and improve your relationship skills and self-esteem. These same steps may prevent an eating disorder from coming back.

Head off a crisis

If you feel depressed and are thinking of suicide, or if you're about to go on a binge or feel like starving yourself, go to the nearest hospital emergency room or call a crisis hot line. Hot lines are listed in the phone book. Contact an eating disorder group and ask for advice. Here is a small list of centers.

- Eating Disorder Referral and Information Center The Eating Disorder Referral and Information Center is dedicated to the prevention and treatment of eating disorders. They provide information and treatment resources for all forms of eating disorders. They also provide referrals to eating disorder professionals, treatment facilities and support groups, etc.
- The 1-800-THERAPIST NETWORK This is a congressionally awarded, international (US and Canada) therapist referral organization.
- National Eating Disorders Association This is a national non-profit organization dedicated to increasing the awareness and prevention of eating disorders.
- Massachusetts Eating Disorder Association, Inc. (MEDA) MEDA's mission is to prevent the continued spread of eating disorders through educational awareness and early detection.
- Anorexia Nervosa and Related Eating Disorders, Inc. This is a nonprofit organization that provides information about anorexia nervosa, bulimia nervosa, binge eating disorder, compulsive exercising, and other less well-known food and weight disorders.
- Aliveness Experience

TREATMENT CENTERS, PROGRAMS

- New Realities Eating Disorders Recovery Centre This site has a good self-assessment questionnaire as well as much useful information.
- Center for Change - Orem, UT A Private Care Center for Women Struggling with Eating Disorders.
- John Hopkins Eating Disorders Program - Baltimore, MD Comprehensive Treatment for Eating Disorders.
- Rogers Memorial Hospital This hospital has specialized residential programming for addictions and eating disorders. This program is unusual in that it treats male patients on an exclusively male unit in a residential setting.
- Monte Nido Treatment Center This is a Residential Treatment Center designed to heal women suffering from Anorexia, Bulimia and Exercise Addiction. Also has a separate unit for males.
- The Renfrew Center
- The Meadows
- Center For Eating Disorders

CHAT, MESSAGE BOARDS

- Chat Support Provides an alternative means of peer support, in a support-group-like format, to individuals suffering with all types of Eating Disorders.

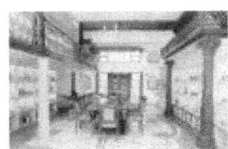

Enroll in a treatment program

Treatment programs offer help with emotions and with healthy eating. You'll learn how to cope with stress, select the right kinds of foods, and exercise safely.

Boost your self-esteem

One-on-one as well as family counseling can help someone with an eating disorder recover fully. Make sure you find a therapist familiar with eating disorders. Be sure to attend your counseling sessions.

As you build trust with your therapist, you'll learn to talk about your hopes and fears about your eating disorder. That will help with your recovery and make stress easier to bear.

Develop a healthy body image

A "good" body doesn't mean one like the thin, ideal bodies you see in ads and on TV. Find out what's healthful and right for you.

Spot and head off stress

Notice which feelings trigger overeating or self-starving. Keep a journal of your feelings. You may find a pattern. Try other ways to ease stress.

Learn to relax. You don't have to be perfect. Take time every day to do something fun just for you. Go for a walk, take a soothing hot bath, or rent a movie. Spend some time every day with a friend or someone in your family who makes you feel at ease. Or call someone who is also trying to recover.

New research is showing that diet soda you're drinking to lose weight may actually be causing you to gain weight instead.

Diet soda may be fizzing with trouble for your waist line. Registered dietician Laurie Meyer, "Diet sodas came into being to help us lose weight and in fact they actually are causing some people to gain weight."

The latest study tracked 1,500 soda drinkers for eight years. In the regular soda group, 47 percent became overweight in that time. In the diet soda group, 57 percent became overweight.

How can that be? Turns out diet soda drinkers are all too often over eaters. They're saving calories in their cup, but they more than make up for it on their plates.

And the more diet soda you drink, the more likely you are to have or develop a weight problem. The pseudo sweet stuff creates real cravings for sweets, and it can change the way your body uses sugar.

The die-hard diet soda fans admit "it's a little scary."

But the good news is, there's a compromise. You can drink one diet soda a day, two tops, along with eating healthy meals, and you should have no trouble.

Research shows that meditation and relaxation exercises can help with stress. Try this meditation exercise:

Sit comfortably in a chair in a quiet place, with your feet flat on the floor and your hands in your lap. Close your eyes and after a minute or so let your mind begin to say a simple phrase or word, sometimes called a mantra. Researchers often suggest the word one. When thoughts come to mind, ignore them and keep returning to your chosen word. Don't feel you have to repeat the mantra all the time; let it come and go. Make it the focus of your energy and attention, but don't focus too hard. After 20 minutes (it's okay to open your eyes to check the time), stop saying the mantra and sit quietly with your eyes closed for a couple of minutes.

Many other exercises can help you relax. Try this one: Slowly tighten and then relax each part of your body, one part at a time: feet, lower legs, upper legs, abdomen, hands, arms, chest, neck, and face.

Many people don't know that there is more safer and effective ways to lose weight.

How much do you weigh? 170 lbs or 210 lbs? We are so self conscious because we are tired of that friend that has the great body getting the most attention. The T.V. shows we watch where our favorite actress weighs 90 lbs.

Exercise, as you well know, is essential for weight loss and overall health. However, many exercisers make mistakes that compromise the effectiveness of their workouts—or worse, increase their risk of injury. Read on to find out if any of these mistakes are getting in the way of your goals.

Not asking enough questions
this is the first place you should start if you are looking into joining a fitness facility or working with exercise professionals. Always check the credentials of your trainers, class instructors, etc. Be sure that any available nutrition information is provided by a registered dietitian.

Inquire about educational background, years of experience, and ask to meet anyone that you may be working with. Aside from making sure that everyone is professionally qualified, it is important to make sure that your personalities are compatible. It is also a good idea to ask the health club's representative about payment options, cancellation policies, whether it is possible to freeze your membership for an extended period of time, etc.

Stop Depression!

Depression is the most common psychological problem in the US. Minor Depression can be attributed to normal depressed feelings that arise because of a specific life situation, a side effect of medication, hormonal changes or physical illness, and do not usually require treatment. Major Depression (depressive illness) is a serious condition that results in extreme fatigue, sleep problems and eventually an inability to function. The exact cause is unknown, but it is thought to be a malfunction of brain neurotransmitters, which are chemicals that modulate moods. Major Depression is usually treated with a combination of psychotherapy and antidepressants which moderate or correct chemical imbalances in the brain. The group of antidepressants most frequently prescribed is the selective serotonin reuptake inhibitors (SSRIs) which regulate the neurotransmitter serotonin.

Get help if you suffer from depression to help conquer weight loss. This is not the main reason for weight gain. But can become part of the problem.

Many things are confusing our choice of how we should look. We all are beautiful in our own ways, but we have a lot of influences telling us we should not look that way in our own skin.

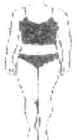

It's no wonder our population is nutritionally deficient. We wouldn't think about putting poor quality fuel in our autos because they would sputter and cough; eventually we'd need a tow truck.

But that's essentially what you're doing if you buy commercial food. What's commercial food you ask? Your typical middle class grocery store.

The average person's state of health is much like a car sputtering and missing a few beats.

If you're buying your food from commercial sources, such as a grocery store, take a look at the difference in the quality of this food versus organic food. Yes, you can starve your body with "empty" or bad food. It's a fact!

The Role of Our Thyroid Gland

Your thyroid is one of your body's most important glands. When your thyroid doesn't work properly, it can cause you to feel nervous or tired; make your muscles weak; cause weight gain or loss; impair your memory; and affect your menstrual flow. A thyroid disorder can also cause miscarriage and infertility.

About 13 million Americans—more of them women—are affected by a thyroid disease or disorder, according to the National Graves' Foundation. In fact, the Colorado Thyroid Disease Prevalence Study suggests that up to one in six people may have an under active thyroid (hypothyroidism).

Women are at least five times more likely to have thyroid dysfunction than are men, but often don't know it. Symptoms often are overlooked or mistaken for symptoms of other conditions. For example, women are at particularly high risk for developing thyroid disorders following childbirth. Symptoms such as fatigue and depression are common during this period, but these symptoms also may be indicators of thyroid disease. More than half of thyroid conditions remain undiagnosed, according to the National Graves' Disease Foundation and the Thyroid Foundation of America. Graves' disease is the most common cause of an overactive thyroid (hyperthyroidism).

The thyroid is a butterfly-shaped gland you can feel at the base of your neck, just below your Adam's apple. Two lobes (the "wings" of the butterfly) fit on either side of your windpipe.

The thyroid gland can be thought of as a manufacturing and storage facility for thyroid hormone (TH), which is often referred to as the body's metabolic hormone. Among other actions, TH stimulates enzymes that combine oxygen and glucose, a process that increases the basal metabolic rate (BMR) and body heat production. TH also helps maintain blood pressure; regulates tissue growth and development; is critical for skeletal and nervous system development and plays an important role in the development of the reproductive system.

The thyroid gland can malfunction in one of three ways:

- It can release too little TH, resulting in a condition known as hypothyroidism (under active thyroid).
- It can release too much TH, resulting in a condition known as hyperthyroidism (overactive thyroid).
- Its tissue can overgrow, resulting in a nodule, a small lump in part of the gland. Most nodules are harmless growths, but small percentages are cancerous. In fact, according to the National Cancer Institute (NCI), tiny and insignificant carcinomas can be found in five to 10 percent or more of all thyroid glands that are carefully examined under the microscope at autopsy, but relatively few of them grow or spread to produce symptoms that lead to their detection during a person's lifetime. The thyroid cancers that are diagnosed each year represent about one percent of all cancers in the U.S. population, according to the NCI.

Hypothyroidism:

When too little TH is released, the body's metabolic rate decreases and the body slows down. Hypothyroidism can go undiagnosed because the following signs and symptoms can easily be mistaken for or attributed to other conditions:

- fatigue
- depression
- low body temperature
- weight gain
- dry or itchy skin
- coarse, dry hair/hair loss
- slow heart rate
- constipation
- poor memory
- trouble with concentration

- hoarseness/husky voice
- irregular/heavy menstruation
  - muscle aches
    - infertility
  - high cholesterol
- goiter (enlarged thyroid gland)

Hypothyroidism can occur spontaneously, develop during or after pregnancy or after treatment for hyperthyroidism. You can be born with it or it can be caused by Hashimoto's thyroiditis, the leading cause of hypothyroidism.

Named for the Japanese health care professional, who first described it in detail, Hashimoto's thyroiditis is an autoimmune disease. Such diseases are characterized by the immune system attacking the body's healthy tissues rather than fighting off invading bacteria or viruses. In this case, the immune system works against the thyroid by producing antibodies to the gland as if it were a foreign substance that needed to be destroyed. The damage caused by the antibodies results in decreased production TH.

Thyroid nodules:

Ranging from as small as a millimeter to as large as several inches, thyroid nodules themselves don't represent illness. In fact, it is estimated that half of the entire population will develop an unnoticeable growth on the thyroid at some time. Nodules do, however, indicate an underlying problem with the thyroid and should be evaluated if they are discovered.

The majorities of nodules are benign and are discrete clumps of thyroid cells, which don't function like normal thyroid tissue. Other nodules turn out to be simple cysts (as shown by ultrasound). However, because there is a slight (five to eight percent) chance that a thyroid nodule is caused by cancer, it is important to have all growths assessed by a medical specialist, according to the American Thyroid Association.

While most nodules are not associated with symptoms, are never detected and are harmless, sometimes they can be large enough to press against the windpipe and cause swallowing difficulty or a cough. An overactive nodule can cause suppression of the rest of the gland and may cause hyperthyroidism.

The thyroid gland is located in the neck just under the Adam's apple. It produces the hormone thyroxin. This hormone is converted outside of the thyroid gland where it becomes activated and stimulates every one of the trillion cells in the body. Almost all of our systems and functions depend upon receiving adequate amounts of this hormone. **The thyroid along with the adrenals is probably the gland most susceptible to the tremendous stress of our fast paced society.** It is the thermostat of the body. It produces hormones that work to keep our metabolic rate stable and keep energy-producing processes in balance. **The thyroid is essential in protein synthesis, growth, temperature regulation, and oxygen consumption of cells.** If the thyroid is depleted or deficient, the rest of the body functions poorly. With low thyroid, cholesterol can shoot up to dangerous levels.

Thyroid disease, both hyperactive and under-active, is so extraordinarily prevalent today that even by conservative estimates it may strike up to 15 percent of the adult population. Women are particularly susceptible, and the disease tends to run in families. A possible reason for the increase in thyroid disease is the high prevalence of auto-immune disease today. Immunity in general is being assaulted by toxic chemicals in food, water, and air. Under-active or hypothyroid conditions can cause low energy.

"Yes" answers to the following questions may indicate a hypothyroid condition.

- Are you depressed, lethargic, and easily chilled?
- Do you gain weight easily?
- Do you suffer from chronic fatigue?
- Do you have dry skin, hair loss, eczema, or adult acne?
- Do you suffer from muscle aches, constipation, and hoarseness?
- Do you have PMS or menstrual abnormalities? Is your libido low?
- Are your feet and legs swollen and your nails brittle?
- Do you get a lot of colds and flu? Low thyroid results in increased vulnerability to infection.

A test may be taken at home to find out if the thyroid is low.
For four days keep a thermometer by your bedside. As soon as you wake up in the morning put the thermometer in your armpit for ten minutes. You must do this before you get up. If you get up first you will not get an accurate reading. If your temperature runs below 97.8 then you most likely have low thyroid. It is important to shake the thermometer after each use.

Some of the common causes of low thyroid, besides inheritance, include: iodine depletion, x-rays or low dose radiation, pituitary and thyroid malfunction, air and environmental pollutants, overuse of diet pills and other drugs, and vitamin A, E, and zinc deficiency.

Treatment for Thyroid Disorder

Avoid refined foods, saturated fats, sugars, and white flour products. If the thyroid problem is severe it is then good to avoid Brussels sprouts, cabbage, broccoli, kale, mustard greens, peaches and pears as they have anti-thyroid substances and may suppress the thyroid function.

Follow a diet with at least 50 % of the foods being fresh, and organically grown to rebalance and establish a better metabolism. The enzymes from live foods help the body to maintain proper metabolism. Foods that heal include sprouts, salads, raw vegetables, and thermos cooked grains to retain enzymes which heal and feed the glands.

Eat foods rich in vitamin A, such as yellow vegetables, eggs, carrots, and dark green vegetables. M.U. Tene is concentrated Beta-Carotene, the precursor to Vitamin A and one of nature's most powerful antioxidants.

Iodine rich foods that nourish the thyroid are: fish and sea vegetables such as: arame, kelp, dulse, hijike, nori, wakame, and Kombu. Seaweeds are very nourishing to the glands.

Zinc and copper are important in helping the body make thyroid hormone. Foods rich in zinc include: beef (range free), oatmeal, chicken (range free), seafood, dried beans, bran, tuna, spinach, seeds, and nuts. Foods rich in copper include: organ meats (range free), eggs, yeast, legumes, nuts, and raisins.

The amino acid tyrosine is helpful. Tyrosine is found in soy products, beef, chicken, and fish.

Black and red radishes have been used by some doctors in the old Soviet Union as accepted medical treatment for hypothyroidism. Raphine, the main sulphur component in radishes, is chiefly responsible for keeping the production of thyroxin and calcitonin (a peptide hormone) in normal balance. Seeds and nuts, seed and nut milks, vegetable juices (celery, parsley, small amount of carrot, Swiss chard, wheat grass) and plenty of green drinks containing chlorophyll for healthy blood are helpful. Earth's Harvest is a blend of three micro-algae's that are a rich whole food source of chlorophyll. Having a mixed vegetable juice that includes the juice of a few radishes, carrot, tomato, celery or zucchini, with a pinch of kelp may benefit the thyroid gland greatly. This juice can be blended in a blender for those who do not have a juicer.

Other beneficial ingredients for vegetable juice combinations include: alfalfa, all leafy greens, beet tops, carrots, celery, green peppers, parsley, seaweeds, sprouts, and watercress.

Diet Pills and Weight Loss

Diet pills are very tempting things if you want to lose weight, especially if you have tried several conventional weight loss diets without success.

Maybe one of your diet buddies has decided to buy diet pills, or maybe you've seen or heard a commercial for diet supplements promising easy fast weight loss.

If so, please beware! Even the most natural-sounding diet pills or weight loss supplements can be useless for weight loss, or dangerous, or both.

Many Diet Pills and Weight Loss Products are Fraudulent

According to *Fat - Exploding the Myths* (Lisa Colles), Americans are reported to spend between $30-50 billion each year on diet and weight loss programs, products and pills; $6 billion of this is said to be spent on weight loss products and pills that are fraudulent.

For an ideal diet to go with your diet pills, **See Anne Collins Diet Program**

Types of Diet Pills - Prescription & Over-the-Counter

We can divide diet pills into two types: prescription-only diet pills and over-the-counter (otc) diet pills.

Prescription Diet Pills

These pills are diet drugs. These pills are regulated by the Food and Drug Administration agency (FDA), their side effects are monitored and they may be advertised and prescribed for weight loss under certain condition and in certain pill-dosages. Examples of prescription diet pills include brands like: Meridia (Sibutramine), Xenical (Orlistat), Adipex, Bontril, Didrex, Phentermine and Tenuate.

Prescription Diet Pills Designed for Obesity Sufferers

Diet pills are principally designed for those suffering from serious obesity - e.g. with a body mass index of 35+. Diet and weight loss drugs are not a cosmetic solution for weight loss, neither are they intended to replace convention diet and weight loss programs. Dieters who fail to lose weight on orthodox diet plans should not turn to pills as an easy answer to their weight problems. Instead they should continue with their weight loss diet and work on improving their motivation to lose weight and exercise.

Over-the-Counter Diet Pills and Weight Loss Supplements

The OTC diet and weight loss pills sector is probably the fastest growing sector of the weight loss industry. However, these diet pills are classified as food supplements rather than diet drugs, and are relatively unregulated. These diet pills are not tested by Federal authorities, not subject to the same advertising, dosage or labeling requirements as prescription diet pills, even though some experts consider that many OTC diet supplements and weight loss pills are (in reality) diet drugs.

Side Effects of OTC Diet Pills Unregulated

Although many CTC diet pills and weight loss supplements contain ingredients with powerful amphetamine-like properties, and even though some of these diet pills have been associated with serious side effects including death, there are no compulsory reporting procedures for these diet products. OTC diet pills remain an unknown quantity.

For an ideal diet to go with your diet pills, **See Anne Collins Diet Program**

The Diet Pills Industry

Most diet drugs companies are trying to invent genuine solutions to the problems of overweight and obesity. They have tried amphetamine-type diet pills, now they are producing diet pills that work on the brain to suppress appetite, or in the gut to inhibit the amount of fat (and calories) digested. And even though prescription-only diet pills are regulated by the Food and Drug Administration agency (FDA), problems persist. In short, like all drugs, diet pills carry health risks.

In addition, as stated above, OTC diet and weight loss pills are becoming more powerful yet remain unregulated. Without doubt, this has allowed certain pill-manufacturers to promote useless, even dangerous diet pills as the solution to weight loss without any evidence to support such weight-loss claims.

Side Effects and Dangers of OTC Diet Pills

The side effects and dangers of OTC diet and weight loss pills can vary enormously because many of these pills contain a cocktail of ingredients and because dosage instructions may be inadequate. Possible side effects include: nervousness, tremor, diarrhea, bulging eyes, racing heartbeat, elevated blood pressure even heart failure.

Side Effects and Dangers of Prescription Diet Pills, Drugs

The dangers of prescription diet pills are consistent with other similar drugs. Accidental overdose is a common problem when taking these diet pills. This is because many diet pills contain similar ingredients to non-prescription medications like nasal decongestants.

Side Effects of Diet Pills That Work on the Brain

Diet pill side effects of drugs that operate on the brain to reduce appetite include: raised blood pressure, chest pain, fever, hair loss, depression, impotence, heart damage, to name a few.

Side Effects of Diet Pills That Work in the Gut

The most popular of the 'gut' prescription diet pills is Xenical. Licensed for long-term use, its side effects include: diarrhea, unexpected fecal discharge and oily stools. To reduce these side effects, Xenical-users are advised to follow a low-fat diet plan.

Are Herbal Diet Pills Any Healthier?

OTC Diet pills with 'Natural', 'Herbal' or similar descriptions are not necessarily any healthier than other diet or weight loss pills. In fact, some of these herbal diet pills are associated with some major health concerns. So don't trust diet pills just because they sound 'natural'.

Do Diet Pills Work?

Yes and No. When used under medical supervision in conjunction with a proper diet and exercise program, diet pills can be effective - at least in the short term. That said, the body adjusts remarkably quickly too many diet pills, so the benefits may quickly wear off.

Diet Pills Are Definitely Not a Magic Solution for Weight Loss

If diet pills are not used in conjunction with a proper weight loss program incorporating proper diet and exercise, they are not likely to be effective. Indeed some pills may even disrupt your system causing weight gain.

Do NOT Buy Diet Pills without Consulting Your Doctor

If you are a genuine candidate for diet pills - i.e. seriously obese, with a will to modify your diet and take regular physical exercise - I strongly advise you to consult your doctor and ask him to explain what weight loss pills may be suitable. Do not buy diet pills without consulting your doctor.

Consulting Your Doctor about Diet Pills

When talking to your doctor about diet and weight loss pills:

- Explain your complete medical history and list all current medications you are taking.
- Ask to be medically examined (blood pressure etc.)
- Ask for an explanation of all your weight loss options.
- Ask for an explanation of all relevant side effects of diet pills suggested.
- Arrange a return appointment to see how the diet pills are working.

Taking Diet Pills

If you decide to take any type of diet or weight loss pills, follow these elementary precautions:

- Take diet pills exactly as prescribed or directed.
- Follow a proper diet and exercise program while taking the pills.
- If side effects persist or worsen, contact your doctor.
- See your doctor after 30 days to discuss your progress on the pills.
- If the diet pills stop working, stop taking them!

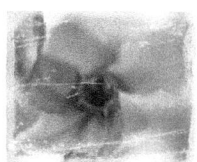

Vitamin/Mineral Therapy

- B-Complex vitamins to help improve cellular oxygenation and energy build the adrenals and the thyroid and calm the nerves. Vita Balance 2000 is a properly balanced, vitamin and chelated mineral complex.
  - Vitamin A assists in maintaining normal glandular function. M.U. Tene is concentrated Beta-Carotene, the precursor to Vitamin A and one of nature's most powerful antioxidants.
- Vitamin C promotes normal adrenal function and glandular activity. Magnum C is an improved form of C known as "Ester C".
- Essential fatty acids are a must for glandular health and they improve over all health. These can be omega 3's and 6's from marine lipids, flax oil or flax seed, black current seed oil, evening primrose oil, or borage oil. New Life 1000 provides essential fatty acids from cold water salmon oil. Life Plus provides essential fatty acids from Blackcurrant Seed Oil.
  - Multi-minerals either liquid or chelated form. All minerals are involved in glandular heath. Vita Balance 2000 is a properly balanced, vitamin and chelated mineral complex. It includes all the trace minerals and an herbal base of related micronutrients.
- Calcium / magnesium, manganese, selenium, silicon and zinc protect the glands. High Grade Calcium Complex provides a microcrystalline form of calcium, plus a balance of associated nutrients necessary for proper calcium assimilation.
  - Iodine supplementation from kelp or dulse, 225 -1,000 micrograms a day.
  - Desiccated natural thyroid, complete with all thyroid hormones. If the symptoms are mild this form may be enough support. If they are severe a synthetic hormone such as thyroxin may be in order.

Herbal Therapy

Irish moss and kelp are used in combination to balance hormonal deficiency. They increase the metabolic rate, thyroid activity and the detoxifying function of the body, and increase blood circulation and soothe inflamed tissues.

Black walnut has a high content of iodine and is a thyroid stimulant.

Ginseng strengthens the body.

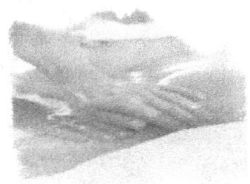

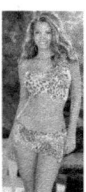

Do you want to look like this? Well we need variety. If every women looked exactly like this. This world would be very boring.

We need meaty women. We need extra skinny women. We need big boned women. Every one needs a lot of guidance to create a secure image for themselves. I found this and thought it was cute.

What Women Want in a Man, Original List (age 22):
1. Handsome
2. Charming
3. Financially successful
4. A caring listener
5. Witty
6. In good shape
7. Dresses with style
8. Appreciates finer things
9. Full of thoughtful surprises
10. An imaginative, romantic lover.

What Women Want in a Man, Revised List (age 32):
1. Nice looking (prefer hair on his head)
2. Opens car doors, holds chairs
3. Has enough money for a nice dinner
4. Listens more than talks
5. Laughs at my jokes
6. Carries bags of groceries with ease
7. Owns at least one tie
8. Appreciates a good home-cooked meal
9. Remembers birthdays and anniversaries
10. Seeks romance at least once a week.

What Women Want in a Man, Revised List (age 42):
1. Not too ugly (bald head OK)
2. Doesn't drive off until I'm in the car
3. Works steady -- splurges on dinner out occasionally
4. Nods head when I'm talking
5. Usually remembers punch lines of jokes
6. Is in good enough shape to rearrange the furniture
7. Wears a shirt that covers his stomach
8. Knows not to buy champagne with screw-top lids
9. Remembers to put the toilet seat down
10. Shaves most weekends.

What Women Want in a Man, Revised List (age 52):
1. Keeps hair in nose and ears trimmed

2. Doesn't belch or scratch in public
3. Doesn't borrow money too often
4. Doesn't nod off to sleep when I'm venting
5. Doesn't re-tell the same joke too many times
6. Is in good enough shape to get off couch on weekends
7. Usually wears matching socks and fresh underwear
8. Appreciates a good TV dinner
9. Remembers my name on occasion
10. Shaves some weekends.

What Women Want in a Man, Revised List (age 62):
1. Doesn't scare small children
2. Remembers where bathroom is
3. Doesn't require much money for upkeep
4. Only snores lightly when asleep
5. Remembers why he's laughing
6. Is in good enough shape to stand up by himself
7. Usually wears clothes
8. Likes soft foods
9. Remembers where he left his teeth
10. Remembers that it's the weekend.

What Women Want in a Man, Revised List (age 72):
1. Breathing
2. Doesn't miss the toilet

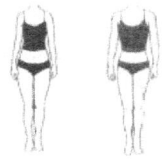

****

Professional Massages are a good stress free program to consider.

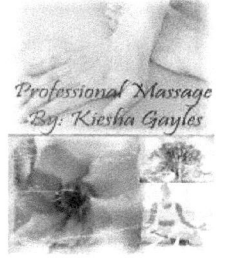
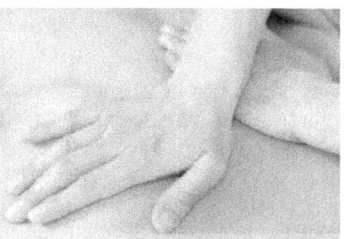

http://www.pmc.iwantamassage.com

http://massagelistings.com/detailsad.asp?ID=430
https://www.massagelistings.com/searchresultsmemb
er.asp

(Massage & Weight)

An alarming 61% of Americans are overweight or obese.[1] In 2001 obesity rates were up 30% since the 1970's and an estimated 1,200 people DIED DAILY from weight-related illnesses.[2] These numbers increase daily. Nearly 10% of our population is diabetic, including many children. And these numbers are modest since many overweight people underestimate their weight.[3] We are a culture of excess. And yet most Americans are on one diet or another. Clearly something is not working.

These statistics are dangerous, and unless our mindset regarding health and fitness undergoes a radical change, we are in for some very unpleasant consequences to our under-active, overfed lifestyles. Unfortunately, most of the diets and weight loss products we use contain ingredients that are toxic to our bodies. This not only prevents most of us from achieving permanent weight loss, but even worse, it prevents us from achieving permanent health. And most of these programs and products do not take into consideration the emotional implications of weight gain. **But all of this can change with the consistent use of therapeutic grade essential oils and more conscious food consumption and exercise.**

What are Therapeutic Grade Essential Oils?

Therapeutic Grade Essential Oils are oils distilled from plants and flowers in a way that preserves as many delicate aromatic compounds within the essential oil as possible. Many factors contribute to the grade of oil – timing, soil, fertilizer used, distillation process. To get the highest quality oil requires time, patience and a commitment to excellence.

There are no regulations in America to gauge the quality of Essential Oils, so picking the right oil is not always easy. Many oils are diluted with solvents to thin the oil, and then synthetic fragrances are added. This process corrupts the oil and can cause rashes, burning and skin irritations, even allergic reactions.

Other oils are misrepresented. For example, Lavender Oil is often not Lavender at all, but a hybrid called Lavandin that is cheaper to produce. It smells nice, but it does not have the same therapeutic value as true Lavender.

While there are no regulations in America, a set of standards has been established in Europe that outlines the chemical profile and principal constituents that quality essential oils should have. These standards are known as AFNOR and ISO (Association French Normalization Organization Regulation and International Standards Organization). They are guidelines that help buyers differentiate between a therapeutic-grade essential oil and lower grade oils with similar chemical makeup and fragrance. Some oils smell nice, but have little value otherwise. Other oils can even be harmful because of what is added. **But Therapeutic Oils can help achieve optimum health and wellness, and even help achieve the perfect weight**. With therapeutic oils you can begin to address all issues of excess weight. Emotional, Hormonal, Physical. Usually we suffer from a combination of problems that contribute to weight gain.

Five Steps to Greater Health

And so, here are five simple ways essential oils can help you lose weight and gain health. Keep in mind, however, that not all oils are created equal. To gain true benefit from essential oils, you should choose the highest quality oils. Many of the products mentioned are from this product line.

1. <u>Deal with the Stress.</u> With our daily lives so full of deadlines, duties and daily chores, we all need to look at the stress in our lives. Often we may eat when what we really need is rest, water, exercise or even just a bath. Look at this issue and ask yourself, "Am I hungry? Or am I just tired? Or thirsty?"

Some oils that can help with stress and bring clarity to these situations include Lavender, the Oil blend "Peace and Calming" and chamomile.

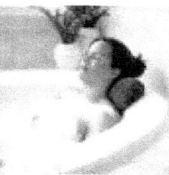

You can apply these to your feet in the morning and at night, and diffuse them in your home throughout the day with a cold air diffuser. If a bath is what you need, then put a couple drops in some bath salts and let the soothing oils soak into your skin. When sleep is the required course of action, put a few drops of your favorite calming oil on a cotton ball and put it in your pillow. However you choose to use the oils, be prepared to feel more relaxed and less inclined to stress eat.

How does it work? Our sense of smell is nearly 10,000 times more sensitive than any of our other senses and it is the only sense directly linked to the limbic lobe of the brain where all of our emotions originate. By applying the essential oil to our body, that connection becomes even more powerful, allowing for true emotional release. These oils have been studied for their therapeutic benefits and have been shown to help relieve symptoms associated with stress and tension.[4]

2. Having trouble controlling your appetite? Try a few drops of peppermint and spearmint in your water. Not only will the water hydrate you and fill your stomach, but peppermint is a natural appetite suppressant and spearmint is great for speeding up the metabolism. A nice side effect is a happier tummy, as peppermint is wonderful for stomach problems. This is also a great substitute for sugary juices and sodas for you and the kids.

Also has three supplements specifically geared for weight loss. ThermaBurn, Thyromin and ThermaMist Oral Spray. These three products together help curb appetite, increase metabolism and give you more energy to aid in weight loss. They are packed with all the essential oils and nutrients necessary to help you accomplish your weight loss goals, and they are safe and healthy for your body.

Balance your hormones naturally. Sometimes weight gain is a byproduct of hormone imbalance. If this is the case for you, try Endoflex. A blend that not only helps balance hormones, but also amplifies metabolism. Put it on your neck and under your big toes three times a day. Just the smell with help create balance. As your hormores become more balanced, those extra pounds won't hang on so stubbornly

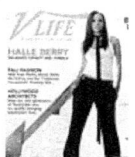

Check out your local store for any magazine.
Many magazines have a lot of info.

Detox. Detox. Detox. Everybody living in our polluted world carries around all kinds of toxins in their systems. These toxins enter us through our food, medications, even the shampoos and lotions we use on our body, not to mention the air we breathe. Your body has to protect itself from these toxins, so it uses fat cells to store them, thus keeping the rest of you relatively safe. If you want to rid yourself of those pesky pounds, you have to put the toxins somewhere else namely out of your body.

The best way to do this is to use a Cleansing Trio. It includes the herbal colon cleanse ComfortTone, the intestinal fiber cleanse ICP and the enzyme cleanse Essentialzyme. Taken for 3 months, these cleansers will go a long way toward flushing out your system and give your body fewer reasons to hold on to extra fat. You can also help this process along by finding a certified healer to give you colonics throughout this process. Remember to drink lots of purified water to help your body flush out the waste and the pounds.

5. Release the Emotional Blocks. Last but not least, we come to the emotional reasons for weight gain. For many of us, it is a coat of protection we wear, for whatever reason. Many people are addicted to the high they get from over-eating their favorite food. Dealing with these issues is essential to keeping the pounds off permanently. Oil Blends has several powerful blends that can help address the emotional issues we all face. "Release", "Present Time", "Hope" and "Harmony" are just a few. These oils can be used in baths, on the skin, with a cold air diffuser or any other way that works for you.

There is a scientific link between what we smell and the parts of our brain that deals with emotions. These oils are powerful stimulants to aid in emotional release, so be prepared for true emotional cleansing. As the emotional baggage is released, don't be surprised to see the pounds go with too. Oil Blends also has an entire kit of oils called the "Feelings Kit" that may be beneficial in helping to target the emotional baggage keeping you overweight.

All of the oils and products recommended here are entirely natural, organic and healthy for your body. They will help aid in the process of weight loss that many of us struggle with. But keep in mind that exercise and diet are essential components in any healthy lifestyle. We all need to exercise our bodies, even if we have no weight problem. And a diet rich in raw vegetables and fruits is important for overall health.

I, personally, have found that a raw vegan lifestyle is most powerful in helping with weight loss and overall health, with the use of these oils as supplements. But everyone must find the lifestyle that fits them best. These oils are tools to help you get where you want to be physically, emotionally, and spiritually.

Types of Diets

Let's take a look at the different diets:

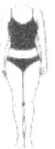

Atkins Diet - Overview

The Atkins Diet is probably the most well known low-carb / high-protein diet. It first appeared back in the early 70's. The Atkins Diet claims you can eat all the protein and fat that you care to and still lose weight. You just need to cut out the carbohydrates to become thin. It's all explained in: *Dr Atkins New Diet Revolution*, by Dr Robert C. Atkins.

One of the Few Genuine Bargains on the Internet

Created by clinical nutritionist and weight loss consultant *Anne Collins*, this online weight management program includes a variety of flexible diet plans to suit most dieters. In addition, it includes a significant amount of advice on diet motivation and exercise, plus a very active weight loss forum. One of our own staff is a member of Collins' program and states that the forum is *"...totally inspirational. Unlike anything I've seen anywhere on the Internet."*

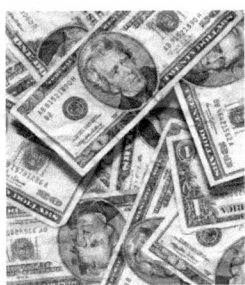

Costs

It costs $19.97 to join the program, and this includes membership of the forum. There are no other fees.
In our opinion this program is **one of the few genuine bargains** on the Internet.

Program Details

- All the diet plans include ordinary foods, plus fast-food options. They seem simple to follow, with a lot of useful information.
- Her weight loss diet-plans include:
  - Low Carb Diet
  - Balanced Diet
  - 14-Day Low Calorie *Booster* Diet
  - GI Diet (For better blood glucose control)
  - Cholesterol-Lowering Diet
  - 10-Minute Meals Diet
  - Vegetarian *Quick-Start* Diet
  - Diet for Life
  - Vegetarian Diet for Life
- Sample menus are given for all diets

- All the diets are available in e-book (PDF) format

  In total there are about 500 pages of information in the diet program to browse or download.

Anne Collins Weight Loss Motivation Advice - "... uncomfortably accurate..."

What is genuinely unique about Collins weight loss program is her advice on motivation. The motivation tips in her program are uncomfortably accurate (but amusing) and you get the feeling she really knows what she is talking about.

In addition, her forum appears to offer exactly the type of personal support which dieters need, but which so few weight loss companies provide.

All this for $19.97? Simply unbelievable.
There are companies offering less than this for $100 or more.

Anne Collins Diet Program - Claims

- Seems easy to follow.
- Convenient meals. Wide range of foods.
- Teaches good eating habits.
- Advice on weight loss motivation.
- No supplements, bars or shakes to pay for.
- 365-Day Customer Support.
- Inspirational Weight Loss forum.
- 12 Months membership costs $19.97. No extras.
- Members receive no spam of any kind.

Anne Collins Diet Program - Drawbacks

- Does not offer 1-800 order numbers.

New Beverly Hills Diet - Overview

The Beverly Hills diet is a food combining diet that relies heavily on fruits. According to the diet, papaya softens body fat, pineapple burns it off and watermelon flushes it out of the body.

Judy Mazel, actress and founder of the diet plan, promises not only that you'll lose weight, but that you'll be "skinny." The problem is she chooses a slightly different way of combining foods - there are days where all you can eat are grapes; on other days you can only have melon.

Introduction
Food intolerance diets are big business. The manufacturers claim that weight gain can be caused by a person's intolerance towards certain foods. By avoiding these foods, weight loss becomes easier.

How it works
Typically, a slimmer pays anything up to $250 and is given a blood test to determine his/her intolerances. Often, the test uncovers a series of such intolerances and the slimmer is then furnished with two separate food-lists - a list of banned foods and a list of permissible foods. The list of banned items frequently contains a wide variety of common foods, including ordinary bread and most dairy products. The manufacturers claim that if the slimmer follows the plan exactly, he/she will lose weight and feel better.

Carbohydrate Addicts Diet Review

Carbohydrate Addicts Diet - Overview:

The basis of the Heller's Carb Addict Diet is that some of us have an addiction to carbohydrates and by controlling them we can ultimately control our weight. It is explained in: *The Carbohydrate Addict's Lifespan Program* - by Rachael Heller & Richard Heller.

At breakfast and lunch you eat meals that include no carbs at all. These meals should be half protein and half non-starchy carbs. For dinner, you have what they call a "reward" meal. This meal should be 1/3 protein, 1/3 carb and 1/3 non-starchy veggies. You can eat for a full hour, but should you choose to have seconds or thirds, you must eat 1/3 protein, 1/3 carb and 1/3 non-starchy veggies. You can't just have the carbs.

Not every celebrity is a natural-born size eight. Some of them actually have to work hard to achieve and maintain their red-carpet-ready figures. So how do they do it?

Undoubtedly, there are some loony diet plans out there with more than one celeb following them; however others stick to sensible and realistic regimes, which achieve great results without sending you gaga. We take eight celebs and show you how to slim like a star.

Until the birth of her daughter Apple, Gwyneth Paltrow famously followed a strict macrobiotic diet plan, which banned all meat, eggs, dairy and caffeine. However, during pregnancy Gwyneth bloomed and she puts the weight gain down to the fact that she ditched the rabbit food and instead indulged her cravings for toasted cheese sandwiches and chips.

Since the baby's arrival, Gwyneth has resumed a healthier eating plan, although she admits she's not as strict on herself as she once was. 'I try to eat as organically as possible and I steer clear of candy because I don't think there's any energy in it,' she says. 'I simply try not to eat any over-manufactured foods that aren't naturally welcome in my body. I try not to eat anything "toxic" that will drain my energy.'

Overview

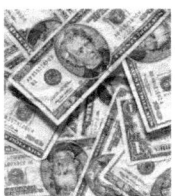

E Diets Program – Cost

EDiets, the market leader in online diets, has a program based around a large diet/food information database. The program offers a wide range of personal diet options so you can personalize your diet plan to suit your preferences. You may also obtain access to a variety of other services, like forums and counseling, although some of these extra weight loss services cost extra.

EDiets Diet Program - Interactive Online Diet Plan

The eDiets web site makes good use of the interactive features of the Internet and the diet advice offered is convenient, realistic and healthy. It caters for all age groups, fitness levels and dietary preferences.

The basic cost for eDiets diet program is $2.99 per week; support services (eg. forum) cost an extra $1.99 per week, adding up to a total of $258 per annum. Check online for latest prices.

EDiets Diet Program - Drawbacks

- The basic cost is not unreasonable, but at around $250 per annum if you want support, it can be expensive. For a lower-priced alternative

Dr Robert Kushner

"Trying to lose weight without knowing your diet personality is like treating hypertension without having first checked your blood pressure."
Dr Robert Kushner

Overview

The resident doctor at www.diet.com is Dr Robert Kushner. Dr Kushner uses his famous diet personality test to assess the dietary and exercise needs of people that need to lose weight.

He is Board certified in nutrition and medicine and has spent many years studying lifestyles and approaches to weight loss and diet. Dr Kushner graduated from the University of Illinois Medical School, Chicago. He also earned his masters degree in clinical nutrition at the University of Chicago.

Often referred to in the media Dr Kushner has appeared on CNN and Good Morning America. Listed in Best Doctors in America is also a note speaker at national and international events on diet and nutrition.

Dr Kushner uses the diet personality test to diagnose the weight and health status of patients before he prescribes a weight loss treatment. In this way he applies very specific solutions for individual overweight clients.

His philosophy is that gaining weight control is more complex than most people think. It is not just about the food that we eat. It is a lifestyle issue. His methods address the many facets of each person's life to bring about long term and sustainable weight loss.

Once he discovers the specific diet personality through the test he then creates

1) Strategies that make it easy to eat the right way without giving up all your favorite foods,

2) Strategies that build up to an exercise routine that is tailored to work in each specific case,

3) Emotional strategies to aid sustainable weight loss.

Each personality specific plan includes a customized two-week quick-start meal plan, food shopping lists, meal substitutes and alternatives to meet most budgets.

Dr Kushner also encourages his weight loss program participants to avail of his group support and diet-buddy facilities

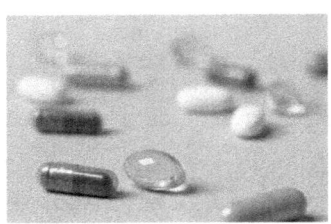

All of these diets have one thing in common. Support system towards losing weight. I think we can lose weight by first curing the need to lose weight for selfish reasons and establish that it is in our nature to move around a lot and start becoming more active. We as Americans are so lazy! Please go out of your way and take out the trash on Wednesday yourself. Walk up to the T.V. and change the channel. If you have a maid gives her a break for a week. Clean your house. While, we are on the subject of cleaning. Did you ever notice that when you clean up you feel great! Why that is because of your endorphins are rising.

Endorphins

Because they are naturally produced by the body, *endorphins* are possibly the best (and most legal way) to achieve a natural high. Chemically speaking, endorphins are *polypeptides*, which able to bind to the neuro-receptors in the brain to give relief from pain. They are one reason why soldiers wounded in battle can continue to fight or have the strength to save someone else; it also accounts for the so called runner's high, or why some people are drawn to dangerous activities like car racing, sky diving and bungee jumping.

While many people are vaguely aware that the blissful feelings one experiences after sex may be endorphin related, few are aware that endorphins are naturally produced by a wide range of activities like meditation, deep breathing, ribald laughter, eating spicy food, or receiving acupuncture treatments or chiropractic adjustments. Fewer still know that endorphins are actually good for health, and can play a role in helping drug and alcohol abusers overcome their addiction. Let's explore some of the dynamics of endorphins and how they affect our daily lives.

What are Endorphins?

First discovered in 1975, endorphins ("endogenous morphine") are one of several morphine-like substances (opioids) discovered within our brains as recently as thirty years ago. Endorphins are polypeptides containing 30 amino acid units. Opioids are considered stress hormones like corticotrophin, cortisol, and catecholamine (adrenaline, noradrenalin), and are manufactured by the body to reduce stress and relieve pain. Usually produced during periods of extreme stress, endorphins naturally block pain signals produced by the nervous system.

The human body produces at least 20 different endorphins with possible benefits and uses that researchers are investigating. Beta- endorphin appears to be the

Endorphin that seems to have the strongest affect on the brain and body during exercise; it is one kind of peptide hormone that is formed mainly by Tyrosine, an amino acid. The molecular structure is very similar to morphine but with different chemical properties.

What do they do?

Although more research needs to be done, endorphins are believed to produce four key effects on the body's mind: they enhance the immune system, they relieve pain, and they reduce stress, and postpone the aging process. Scientists also have found that beta-endorphins can activate human NK (Natural Killer) cells and boost the immune system against diseases and kill cancer cells.

Are endorphins related to the famous "runner's high"?

In contrast to short-intensity workouts like sprinting or weightlifting, prolonged, continuous exercise like running, long-distance swimming, aerobics, cycling or cross-country skiing appears to contribute to an increased production and release of endorphins. This results in a sense of euphoria that has been popularly labeled the "runner's high."

You eat too much. ``How could I have finished that entire pizza?" ``That steak cried out, `Eat me!'''. When what goes in exceeds what you burn, your body has left-over nutrients floating around in the bloodstream.

We evolved in a world where the normal conditions of life were hunger and cold. On those rare occasions the body enjoyed a feast it, like the prudent squirrel, made provisions for the hard times that would surely follow.

Fat cells are the body's equivalent of a piggy bank. Fat cells sit on the banks of the bloodstream and, whenever they see excess food, snatch it out and build molecules of fat to stuff in their little cellular storehouse. Each fat cell is, in essence, a little rubber bag: when it sees too much food it snarfs it up and expands.

When this goes on, the larger rubber bag expands: you gain weight.

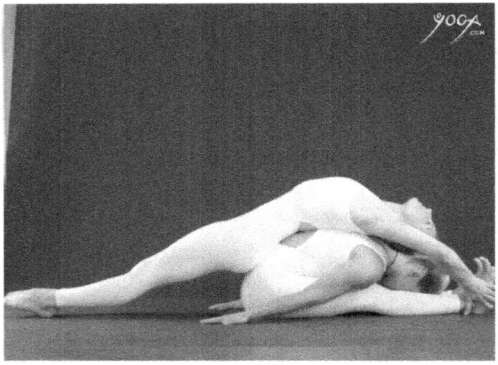

Pain/Endorphines

It also may contribute to what some athletes call a "second wind." Rather than feeling pain and exhaustion while running, endorphins may help us actually feel limber and energized towards the end of a race. According to William Straw, M.D., a team physician for the San Jose Sharks, "at some point you may feel a little more energetic and you can kick-in when you did not feel like you could kick-in before."

Q: Is a prescribed amount of exercise needed before endorphins are released?
A: Endorphins release varies according to the individual: one runner may have an endorphin rush (experienced as a second wind) after running for ten minutes, while another may need to run for thirty minutes before feeling a second wind.

Things to consider

Controlling your weight provides an interesting window on the enigma of sentence, the distinction between mind and body. Weight control involves the body at the simplest level; eat more and gain weight, eat less and lose it. Yet the reasons we become overweight and the difficulties we have in losing weight often stem from the subtleties of psychology rather than the mechanics of mitochondria.

To control your weight, you need only eat the right amount. To eat the right amount, not just this month or next month, but for the rest of your life, you need not only the information--the display on the face of the eat watch--to know what's the ``right amount''; you need an incentive to follow that guidance. Wearing a watch doesn't make you a punctual person, but it provides the information you need to be one, if that's your wish.

This incentive is the ``motivation to control your weight,'' often simplistically deemed ``will power.'' Where can you find this motivation, especially if you've tried diet after diet and failed time after time? This book will help you to find the motivation in the only place it can be found, within yourself, by laying out a program that makes the steps to success easy and the thought of failure or backsliding difficult to contemplate.

This constitutes manipulation, but manipulation's OK as long as you're manipulating yourself. After all, in order to manipulate somebody you have to understand them and who do you understand better than yourself? The goal is empowerment: the sudden realization, ``Hey, this isn't hard at all! I can do this!'' It is such discoveries that give us the confidence and courage to go onward to greater challenges. The course of a life is often charted by such milestones of empowerment. Manipulation in the pursuit of empowerment is no vice.

Latent within you is the power to control your weight for the rest of your life. All you need to do is realize that your weight is under your conscious control. With that knowledge, you can peel off your excess weight and achieve physical fitness. Once you've accomplished those goals, you'll be in a position to make them central to your self-image.

Less than 12 months from now, new people you meet will be incapable of imagining you as overweight. Next year, you'll be able to run up four flights of stairs and scarcely notice the exertion. If, like me, you've been overweight most of your life, you're about to partake of a new and rich part of the human experience: the exultation of living in a healthy animal body.

Once you've experienced the joy, the confidence, and the feeling of power that success entails, you'll never consider giving it up--not even for that extra slice of pie.

Taking your calcium pills 2 times a day. Running at least one hour a day. Women can use strip aerobics for more fun exercise program. Teri Hatcher, Lucy Liu, Christina Applegate, Jennifer Love Hewitt and even *Bachelor* Bob Guiney are already devotees. Carmen Electra and Sheila Kelley liked it so much that they launched their own versions of the exercise: Aerobic Striptease DVDs (AerobicStriptease.com) and The S Factor classes in Los Angeles (SFactor.com), respectively. But the man who's credited with starting it all is Jeff Costa, who, after being a stripper, a choreographer and an aerobics teacher, decided to put it all together and create the Cardio Striptease (CardioStriptease.com) workout and DVDs for Crunch gyms worldwide.

With moves like the "BLT," which stands for breast, leg and thigh; the "Hello Kitty," a full squat to the floor with your feet together but knees spread; the "California Roll," a pivot and grind move; and "Spicy California Roll," like the regular roll with your arms overhead, it's clear this isn't your mother's Jane Fonda workout. Men can sit on the floor and do sit-ups. Hey if you are in shape your sex life will become better!

Eat your green vegetables, lots of salmon, organic foods!

Take your vitamins-Folic acids, fish oil, calcium, vitamin C & D.

There is no magic secret to losing weight and keeping it off, just as there is no hidden key to instant wealth. Nonetheless, every year another crop of ``magic diet'' and ``secrets of investing'' books appear on already-creaking shelves. The human capacity to ignore inconvenient facts and avoid unpleasantness is immense. Success in any endeavor requires coming to terms with the true nature of the task at hand and, if the goal is worth the effort, getting on with it.

``How can I lose weight?'' ``Simple, *eat less food than your body burns*.'' Vitamin C supplements and walking up and down your stairs. Will start your metabolism towards burning fat!

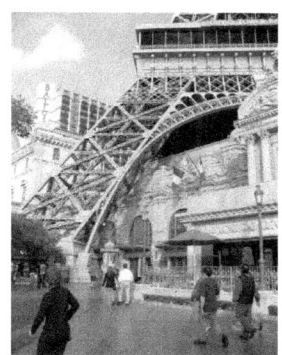

Live an extended life!

Author: Kiesha Gayles

www.ingramcontent.com/pod-product-compliance
Lightning Source LLC
Chambersburg PA
CBHW071309280526
45788CB00004B/1868